SEX POSITIONS

YOUR DEFINITIVE GUIDE FOR A SPICY RELATIONSHIP

MARK G.MOORE

TABLE OF CONTENTS

INTRODUCTION 3

CHAPTER ONE 9

REASONS YOU OUGHT TO BRING IN SOME FUN SEX POSITIONS TO YOUR SEX LIFE 9

CHAPTER TWO 42

THE PROS AND CONS OF THREE SEX POSITIONS 42

CHAPTER THREE 69

SEX POSITIONS TO TRY FOR FUN AND PLEASURE 69

CHAPTER FOUR 91

THE BEST SEX POSITION 91

CHAPTER FIVE 100

ADVANCED SEX POSITIONS 100

CHAPTER SIX 114

BEST SEX POSITIONS FOR ORGASM 114

CHAPTER SEVEN 135

THE BEST SEX POSITIONS TO KEEP PREGNANCY AWAY 135

CHAPTER EIGHT 151

ORAL SEX POSITIONS 151

CONCLUSION 189

INTRODUCTION

Love making is considered to be an art which requires practice. To increase your sex-appeal and to satisfy your partner's desire you need to explore new techniques of making love and experiment with new sex positions. The more you educate yourself, the more you gain confidence in your performance. Each couple has different goals for satisfaction and containment and they have different demands. Before you go for the selection of the best sex positions you need to know your partner's demands. The definition of satisfaction actually depends on various individual components which vary for different peoples. Even the demands of both the partners change in every session that they enjoy.

The body type of every individual is different from the other one. The flexibility and stretching ability of human body differ from one another. Strength in the muscles and bones and energy level are the other factors which you need to consider while selecting the lovemaking positions for yourself.

Preferences are different for every individual. Your partner might want you to be wild in bed; however, you might want to go for a slower and erotic lovemaking session. Both of you need to be at the same page before you start.

Understanding and mood are the two prime factors which need to be taken care of before you indulge. There are people who need no have an emotional relationship with their partner before they start making love. You need to respect those feelings of your partners and give some space for preparation.

The best sex positions

There are thousands of sex positions practiced in different countries by different couples. Everyone differs from one another. As discussed earlier, you need to practice to become perfect. Experimentation is always advised in these cases. Education and awareness will help both of you to gain perfection. You can sit together and explore all the possible lovemaking positions and you will get the best from them. Exploration of sex positions does not mean watching porn movies. It is a proper education and you might download the pages from the different websites. You and your partner need to agree on the selected position according to your body type, energy level, and flexibility. Otherwise, you might get hurt while trying to perform in a tough position like the wheelbarrow.

Hundreds of videos and pictures of best lovemaking positions are available on the internet. The only thing you need to do is download them and learn the proper position for the ultimate pleasure.

CHAPTER ONE

REASONS YOU OUGHT TO BRING IN SOME FUN SEX POSITIONS TO YOUR SEX LIFE

Intimacy is a vital element to any long-lasting romantic relationship. One usual factor as to why breaks up take place is that the partners fail to sustain their sexual intimacy. Sex is something that is able to nurture both the soul and the body. In order to always keep the sexual aspect of your relationship active, you should think of trying some fun sex positions from time to time. Listed here are 4 reasons why.

1. It can put the spice back in a relationship. Adding fun to sex is a really good cure to monotony in the relationship. And just what better method to add fun into sex than to try creative and new positions? You see, when you are doing the same things repeatedly, sex comes to be a routine. If sex becomes routine, it is easy for boredom to set in. When you let an unfulfilling sex life rule your

relationship, you will find yourselves drifting away from each other. Adding fun to sex is a resolution that can stop boredom and sustain the intimacy in your relationship.

2. It can accentuate your climax. If you want to experience this yourself or make your partner orgasm and you are finding it challenging with your usual sexual encounters, then you might just wish to try a few new fun sex positions. These positions are useful in making your partner, in particular when it comes to

the female, reach a climax and have an incredible orgasm. Position matters whenever it comes to bringing your partner to bliss.

By tweaking some of your basic sex positions the fun can really kick off. Using precise targeting of the g-spot by means of the right positions, you and your partner can expect to have the most extraordinary sex ever.

3. It may reduce your stress. Being stuck in a sex routine could add to a stressful relationship. It would not do you or your

loved one any good to have sex when either of you feel that it is an obligation. This turns into a different story with fun sex positions. By breaking the dullness of sex, these sorts of positions may add exhilaration and bliss to intercourse.

When you look forward to undertaking something that provides you so much pleasure, it can help your body produce and release hormones that can minimize your stress levels. If you want to ease any tension in your relationship and restore the spice, try and deviate from your typical sex positions and try out some fresh and unfamiliar ones.

4. Live a much longer life. With the three previous reasons, trying fun sex positions will help you as well as your partner live a longer life. Statistics reveal that sex in itself has the potential to strengthen your body's natural protection against illnesses and diseases. Added to this are the benefits you can get from fun and laughter such as healing and delaying the aging process.

These four are good justifications for you to see sex from a different point of view. By doing this, you can open yourselves to numerous positions that may bring more pleasure and gratification to you and your partner. Perhaps it's time you engage and benefit from some fun sex positions?

The Basic of Sex Positions

Sex has and probably always will be a taboo subject; however, it is entirely natural and is something that the large majority of us will experience at some point in our lives. Obviously, each sexual experience that you have will be unique, but there are some basic sexual positions that are accepted as being the 'industry standard'. Some of these will be discussed in this part but first, there is a small warning......be safe

Everyone seems to go on about this but it is so, so important to wear protection when having sex, particularly with a new partner. With so many STDs and STIs that do not have visible symptoms, it is easy to be too trusting and risk infection yourself. Without going on about it, the best advice is simply not to take the risk.

BEGINNERS SEX POSITIONS

There are several sex positions that apparently belong in the beginners' category. This is not to say that these positions are any less enjoyable than those that are said to be 'expert' positions and in fact many of the following positions regularly top polls for people's favorite positions.

1. The missionary position

The missionary position is probably the single most common sexual position used by couples across the globe. It involves the man lying on top of the woman facing down, whilst she faces up towards him. This is a particularly intimate sexual position.

2. Woman on top

This position does exactly what it says on the tin. The man lies on his back with the woman on top of him, normally on her knees with her shins touching the ground and facing her partner. Many women enjoy the element of control they get with this position - they are able to dictate the tempo and angle of penetration.

3. Doggy style

Borrowed from our canine companions this position involves the woman on all fours with the man penetrating her from behind whilst holding onto her bum or sides. The lack of face to face contact can be an issue for some, but doggy style remains one of the most popular sexual positions.

4. 69er

The 69 or 69er is an oral intercourse position and allows the man to pleasure the woman, whilst she pleasures him at the same time. Either partner can go on top, or you can attempt the position side-on.

A healthy sexual relationship involves experimentation. Talk to your partner about what you are and aren't comfortable doing and what you would like to try. Don't feel pressured into doing something that you are not happy with and above all, enjoy yourself.

SEX POSITIONS THAT FOCUS ON HER PLEASURE

All women love the closeness and intimacy that comes with relationship sex. Here we look at the best sex positions that focus on her pleasure.

1. Missionary sex

Like coming home, always in fashion and like the perfect hand fitting the perfect glove. Everyone will always do missionary. For the woman that loves to be penetrated with the added romantic connection of skin to skin touch, with the ability to kiss, caress and move together. Let your man dominate in these sensuous couples making love positions by controlling the pace and the depth while thrusting your hips up to match his, causing friction and the onset of orgasm. Squeezing and contracting your vaginal muscles in this position is also a great bonus for your partner.

2. Starfish position

A variation of missionary where the man spreads his legs out wide like a starfish and the woman closes hers to allow for extra vaginal tightness and better clitoral stimulation. Other variations include the woman wrapping her legs around her partner's waist, or over his shoulders which can be assisted with a pillow under her buttocks, allowing for deeper penetration.

If you can't orgasm alone with this position, try different variants which will allow your partner to touch your clitoris directly while thrusting.

3. The figure eight

This is a hot, sensual variant of missionary and one of the best couples making love positions! As you lay back with your legs half bent wide open, your partner is positioned at a higher angle than ordinary missionary with his hands by your head. Relax and let the incredible sensation take over as he makes slow, sexy, circles or figure eights. You will be taken to another level as this dreamy movement stimulates your whole vagina and his pubic bone lightly rubs your clitoris. As he maintains this tantalizing movement and also gives you sensual kisses, your body will shudder with an all-encompassing full body climax.

4. The love seat

So 60's, so sensual and intimate with a difference. This position is perfect in a big bean bag while watching a sensual movie. Here you are in command. Slowly move your rear up and down at a pace you decide. You can both add some light sensual touching, he rubbing your back and buttocks and you reaching down to play with his balls.

5. The face forward grind

One of the most intimate, beautiful couples making love positions. Sit on your partner face first with your legs wrapped around his waist while he also sits upright crossed legged. The allure of this upright position is that it allows for long sensuous kissing and touching of each other's faces while being able to look each other directly in the eye.

Gently grind and enjoy a softer, loving, sexual experience.

6. On bended knee

Kneel facing each other with you placing one leg over his thigh. Then let the titillation begin as you rock back and forth as your breasts jiggle and brush his chest. You will love it for the close face to face contact. Give him long kisses and tickle his balls for greater pleasure.

COUPLES MAKING LOVE POSITIONS

7. Cradle sex position

This position has so many advantages. Have your partner kneel in front of you. Facing him position your legs on either side of his hips. Lower yourself on to his penis, then lean back placing your hands behind you. This position offers excellent visuals for him with your beautiful body stretched back before him, and the extra ego boost of seeing his manhood thrust in and out of you. He can also lean forward to lick and tease your nipples or force deeper thrusting with his hands grabbing your buttocks. Start by sitting on him upright with your arms around him for balance. Look him in the eye and rub his manhood up and down your whole vagina to warm you up. Then when you can't take it any longer slip him inside and let him take charge as you lean back.

8. Butterfly position

Relax and fly like a butterfly in this low maintenance position for you. Lay back on the edge of the bed with your partner standing in front of you with your legs over his shoulder at approximately a 45-degree angle. From here you can comfortably lay back as he lifts your hips at your buttocks for the optimal angle of thrusting. If penetration alone does not work for you in the butterfly position, he can also stimulate your clitoris or anus to reach climax.

9. Scissors sex position

This position will certainly take you on a whirlwind ride for you both. Lay on the edge of your bed or table with your man standing in front of you holding your legs up. As he plunges in and out, he alternates opening your legs out wide to shut and crossed back over. Your vagina will be saturated with sensations from profound penetration to a tight snug fit and the possibility of rippling orgasms.

10. 69 sex position

The 69 is one of the most popular lovemaking positions as earlier discussed. It is excellent for sumptuous, mutual suction. Suck away, wriggle or move slightly back and forth. Shift from his penis to balls or anus. And for those high achievers out there, with practice, you can even go for simultaneous orgasm.

11. Sideways 69 sex position

Another one of those hot, tantalizing lovemaking positions, the sideways 69 allows for different angles for optimal suction on each genital area while giving your neck a break from the regular 69. It's also hot to have each other's arms wrapped around your waists and buttocks, pulling you eagerly to each other while moving in a sensual rhythm.

12. Spoons sex position

The spoons sex position is good if you're feeling a little lazy. Lay on your side with your hand resting on your head, the mattress on the bed will help with the rocking motion of him thrusting you back and forth. There's not a lot of work required of you at all. But if you want extra stimulation, have you or your partner rub your clitoris.

TIPS FOR COUPLES

Many couples become quite unadventurous in their sex life as their relationship matures. This is a shame because the key to ensuring your sex life remains active and healthy is to introduce some variety. The Kama Sutra and other sex 'manuals' have popularized the idea of different sex positions, but many people are daunted about trying something new. Here are some tips to make sex positions more enjoyable and more varied:

A variation on the well-known missionary position is for the woman to lie on her back with the man lying beside her facing her. He then enters her with their legs entwined. This has the great advantage of allowing the man to lie down if is not feeling too full of energy while still entering the woman from a very pleasurable angle. It also allows room for the man (or woman) to stimulate the clitoris at the same time. The couple can still maintain eye contact and physical closeness.

If the man is much heavier than the woman this can also be a lot more pleasant for the woman.

In the doggy position (where the woman is kneeling while the man enters from behind), the pleasure for the man can be greatly enhanced if the woman reaches underneath to stroke his testicles. The man can also lean over and play with the woman's breasts.

The man can also use his hands to stimulate the woman's anal area, as well as her inner thighs and clitoris. So the key to doggy style is - use your hands!

When the woman is lying on top of the man, a lot of men get intense visual pleasure from the sight of the woman's breasts. If you are the woman, vary the angle of your chest to give different angles for visual and physical stimulation. Lean down and allow your breasts to lightly touch his chest.

Lean back, and even sit upright so he can see and massage your breasts. He will love it! The man should use the opportunity to really explore the woman's body; don't forget her arms and buttocks, both very sensitive areas.

If any position hurts or is in any way uncomfortable, stop. Always ensure you have sufficient lubrication, but if this is the case and it is still unpleasant it is probably due to the angle of penetration.

Not every woman's vagina is exactly the same shape so don't feel bad to say so if hurts you.

The three positions described above - missionary, doggy and woman on top - are the most popular for couples, and for a reason: they provide the most pleasure. Other 'exotic' positions may look good in photographs or porn films but they not be as easy to achieve as they look. However, just within the three main sex positions, you can achieve a lot of variety through different angles.

The key is to experiment. If it doesn't work well for you at least you can smile about it together. Experimenting and trying new things is all part of the fun.

CHAPTER TWO

THE PROS AND CONS OF THREE

SEX POSITIONS

Well, in this part, I'd like to focus your attention on three popular sex positions and, in particular, the advantages and disadvantages of each one. We will be considering the missionary position, the "man-standing-up-woman-lying-down" position and the woman on top position.

1. Missionary position

This is the traditional position for sex where, as I'm sure you know, the man lies down on top of a prone woman for intercourse.

Pros

This is the easiest sex position to get into, requires little energy to get started and is great for sudden, spontaneous, unplanned sex. It is generally easy for the man to just roll over on top of the woman and their genitals are right opposite each other. This position lends itself to great intimacy because the two lovers can hug each other and look into each others' eyes (if they are roughly the same height). Intercourse feels very exciting for the man, and the woman gets to receive some significant thrusting and a "whole body" experience.

It is usually fairly quiet and can be done secretly if there is a danger of being discovered by other people in the house.

Cons

This position has a reputation for being the "boring, married-people type of sex" since it tends to lend itself to passionless "quickies" and can be repeated every time a couple have sex. It is often resorted to in order to avoid being discovered by curious kids and other people who might interrupt the session. The high levels of stimulation often because the man to ejaculate quickly in less than 2-3 minutes, creating a bad habit for his body and a boring experience for the woman, whose body has hardly begun to respond to the sex before it's all over. It is challenging for the man to create an orgasm for his woman unless he spends a LOT of time in foreplay beforehand and even then, lengthening the time having intercourse is quite difficult.

2. Man standing up, woman lying down

This is the position where the woman lies down with her hips aligned with the edge of the bed, while the man stands up at the edge of the bed for intercourse.

Pros

The main advantage of this position from the man's point of view is the fact that it dramatically lengthens the amount of time he can have intercourse with the woman - anything up to 10-20 minutes or more can be achieved. Having sex standing up makes it much harder for his body to be stimulated to orgasm, so he has to thrust for a longer time to achieve it. He can also see the woman's body much better and can use his hands to touch her breasts and upper body, which allows the woman to receive stimulation in two different ways at the same time. The woman usually holds her legs wide open by placing her hands behind her knees. He can also watch his penis slide in and out of her, the sight of which is a major turn-on. He can also thrust much deeper, so he can reach the woman's A-spot, which can give the woman "cervical" orgasms.

Cons

Having sex comfortably while standing up requires that the bed be at the same height as the man's hips. Usually, it isn't - it's lower. This means that the man has to bend at the knees to be able to have intercourse with the woman. This is tiring on the man's legs because he has to thrust for a long time, plus there is the issue of his bent knees meaning that his legs are not flush with the edge of the bed. This can be resolved by pulling the woman's hips off the bed, so that the small of her back is on the edge of it, but this requires that the woman change the position of her legs by folding them up against her chest in order to counteract the centre of gravity, so her whole body doesn't slide off the bed - in which case, she will end up sitting on the floor with her legs wide open. Folding her legs up against her chest means that the man is no longer able to access her breasts and upper body, so that avenue of stimulation is closed off. Inexperienced women may not realize that they need to hold their legs open with their hands behind their knees and so they will dangle their legs off the end of the bed past the man's body, which can be uncomfortable. There is a greater risk of injury to the woman's vaginal tissues from heavy thrusting since the man can go deeper.

3. Cowgirl position

This is the position where the woman gets on top of a prone man and straddles his hips for intercourse.

Pros

This position is a winner in many ways - it feels awesome to the woman and is extremely exciting for the man. The main benefit is for the woman - she can control everything that is going on and do exactly what she needs to do to achieve an orgasm without relying on the man's expertise and experience. She can do exactly what feels good to her, whether or not he knows how to do that or not. She can go deep or shallow, fast or slow, in and out, up and down, she can rock back and forth, grind her pelvis against his pubic bone for clitoral stimulation, lean backwards, lean forwards, lean left and right, sit facing the man, do "reverse cowgirl", sit on the left of his body, sit on the right, go around and around like she's sitting on a swivel chair and all kinds of stuff! For the man, he gets to watch his woman having the time of her life doing whatever she wants to get the maximum pleasure she can out of his body, which is a major turn-on for him and, secretly, giving his woman a totally mind-blowing time is what every man wants, and this is the lazy way to achieve it without him having to learn any "skills". However, learn he will, since watching her is highly educational and he will find out exactly what turns her on without having to "try everything and watch her carefully to see what happens", which is the usual method of approach for us guys. She can teach her man a lot in a short time and he can remember it all for the next time he's in control. In the meantime, he can lay back and enjoy the ride as much as her because his penis gets lots of stimulation. He can also use his hands to stimulate her breasts and upper body, run his fingers through her hair, tilt her head back and many other things. In addition, there is the reversal of dominance - putting the woman in control of the sex is liberating for her and wildly exciting for him, as he discovers just how much of a wild girl his woman really is.

Cons

This position is high energy for both partners. That could also be a plus, but for the woman, her legs need to be really strong to cope with all the up and down movement, which needs to go on more or less nonstop for at least 20 minutes for her to achieve an orgasm. It is a major cardiovascular exercise and feat of physical endurance. There will be sweat and slippery bodies and a lot of heavy breathing and noise. It is quite stimulating for the man and there is the risk of early ejaculation, ending it all rather quickly before he's had a chance to learn anything or see things really heat up, although women naturally tend to grind more than slide up and down, which can delay his orgasm quite well. His penis needs to be hard for this - he needs a strong erection and it needs to last a long time. There is also a risk of damage to the penis if the girl is really forceful in dropping her whole upper body weight on top of it and she misses her vagina (ouch!) There can be bending of the penis in this case, which is quite a serious injury (often requiring hospitalization!) Also, achieving entry of the penis into the vagina at the beginning can be a little difficult, since the man's penis is pointing upwards and is flat against his body, so either he has to move his penis to a 90-degree position to his body (the usual way) or else she has to lean forward quite a bit for him to put it inside her. There is the also the risk of the noise being detected by other people around, so choose a quiet time for this, when there are not many people around!

So these are the advantages and disadvantages of these three sex positions. If you are considering spicing up your sex life with some new positions, I hope this information helps you to choose the one you want, so that both of you can achieve an exciting and amazing sex life together!

HOW TO HAVE THE BEST SEX EVER?

Everyone asks themselves what are the sex positions for the best sex ever. We want to please our partner when we are making love. So to have the best sex ever it is important that you try sex positions that make intercourse fun and exciting.

Society has a misconception that men should be thrusting deeply into a woman like a jackhammer, while women should be moaning in pleasure nonstop. This happens often in romantic movies but rarely in real life.

One problematic attitude that comes from films is that sex begins and ends when the man comes. Usually, that is considered the climax of making love. The problem with this is that it completely ignores whether women reach orgasm during intercourse.

The truth is that men come quickly, while women hardly ever come. Do not take this as a threat to your manhood.

What this does mean is that one should not treat sex in terms of whether you come or not but whether she can. The difference is sometimes as simple as using different forms of arousal. For example, it is important to stimulate a woman during foreplay and sex with your fingers and penis to get her turned on.

This gives her a prolonged experience and warms her up to be able to orgasm in the first place. Unlike men, women's arousal happens more gradually and is built up by anticipation. Thus doing this stimulation should not just be thought of as incidental, but as something that can make sex last longer and result in more orgasms.

If a girl still does not come, you may want to try something different. For example, if you want a woman to come during vaginal intercourse, try a new sexual position. There are very practical advantages to this. Different positions arouse her in different ways. In fact, simply sitting up or lying on top of her can change the effect dramatically. Making love in various positions adds variety that can keep her more excited. Some positions actually help sex last longer so she can have more orgasms and you can feel like a stud.

Here are some sex positions for the best sex ever. For best results, I strongly recommend warming her up first by stimulating her with your finger so that she gets excited about this. That alone will create more orgasms and skyrocket the times that she reaches her climax. Get your fingers wet and enter her and curve your fingers upwards. Do it slow then speed up. With your other finger rub her clit and lick it with your tongue. This stimulation will get her so excited. When you enter her, you have tried sex with the woman on top. Doing this allows her to move at her own pace and to adjust the angle and depth of penetration. The added advantage of this is that it also allows for more clitoral stimulation that is likely to turn her on. Often she will prefer slow lovemaking, but just as often she will enjoy entering you hard. I want to add one word of caution for both of these positions. I strongly recommend holding her hips to guide them just in case she gets too enthusiastic, which can have painful consequences.

Once you've experimented with these sexual positions, you might try entering her from behind and rub her clit at the same time. This can get her incredibly aroused. You can even, if you time it right, both achieve orgasm at the same time. One of the other great elements of this sex position is that going from behind shows a lot of dominance that psychologically appeals to many women. I would recommend coming up with your own variations as well. You can even try wilder and crazier stuff like thrusting into her while standing up in the shower!

Finally, I would like to add that any one of these sex positions can be varied in other ways as well. For example, looking at her in the eyes while you do any of these adds intensity to making love. Sometimes pinning her arms down while in a missionary position will show dominance that might turn her on. Slowing down your movements and letting her feel each thrust adds more of a sensual, romantic mood that you can sometimes contrast with faster thrusting at other times. By throwing in these new moves and variations you may find her reaching orgasms more often than you've ever seen before

CHAPTER THREE
SEX POSITIONS TO TRY FOR
FUN AND PLEASURE

Sex is one area of your life that you definitely want to ensure has variety to keep it from going stale. Even simple variations on your favorite positions can enhance your pleasure and fun. Here are another 6 sex positions that you might not have thought of. You might like to try to see what you think!

1. Woman lying flat on her stomach with man on top.

This is a variation of the familiar 'doggy' position except the woman is lying flat rather than being on her knees. the man lies on top of here, also flat although using his elbows for support. This is a wonderfully sensuous position. It allows the man to feel the entire length of the woman's body, including being able to kiss her neck. It can also give the woman a feeling of being totally under the man's control which for many women, in the right situation, can be erotic in its own right.

This is a great position for when the two of you are not feeling particularly energetic for sex. It can be a wonderful way to make love late at night, just before sleep.

2. Woman sitting on man facing away. This is very visually exciting for the man as he gets a good view of the woman's buttocks and anus.

He could also tickle her anus lightly while in this position. If the woman puts the weight on her knees, the man can control the penetration with his hips, and also by holding the woman's hips with his hands. The woman can lean slightly forward, which will put added pressure to the base of the penis and the back wall of her vagina.

3. Woman lying on her back, man lying on side with one of her legs between his. Again, a very visual position for the man, as he is also able to see his penis moving in and out of the woman. Man is also able to stimulate the woman's clitoris in this position.

This is something of a variation on the standard 'missionary' position but is a bit more restful for the man.

4. Couple standing with man behind and the woman leaning forward. Make sure the woman has something firm to lean on, such as a bed or wall. this can be great for a 'quickie'!

5. Woman lying on back with a cushion underneath; man kneeling in front between woman's legs. This raises the woman's hips, allowing the man to penetrate at a different angle to the

normal 'missionary' position. Again, it is a very visually exciting position for the man.

6. Lying side by side with man behind. Sometimes called 'spooning' but this involves actual penetration rather than just cuddling. The woman may lean forward slightly to gain a better angle of entry.

Varying the sexual positions used in a relationship can do a lot to keep your love life exciting and fresh. Of course, the traditional favorites such as missionary and doggy positions are wonderful, but experiment with these positions described above and other positions, and communicate with your partner about what each of you likes the best.

SEX POSITIONS YOU'D BE CRAZY NOT TO TRY!

Tired of the same old sex positions? Want to add a little spice to your love life? Try these 5 crazy sex positions with your lover tonight!

1. The dragon position

In this sex position, the woman stretches out onto her stomach, with her legs slightly apart, placing a few pillows underneath her pelvis to raise her buttocks. Her partner can then easily penetrate her by stretching over on top of her. It's a great alternative to traditional rear entry position, offering deep penetration and relief to people who suffer from knee problems.

2. The butterfly position

This is one of the best sex positions for women because it positions the man in such a way as to give easy access to her g-spot. So no matter how he moves, her favorite pleasure spots will always be stimulated. In this position, the woman lies on her back, while the man elevates her hips with his arms to align both of their genitals. He can then move, freely in all directions, alternating as he watches her growing sexual desire

3. Reverse cowgirl position

In this sex position, the woman faces her partner's feet while she sits astride him. She has the control in this position, which allows her the freedom to move at the rate and speed that fills her to brink of pleasure. Her man, laying beneath her can either relax and enjoy the rear view or move in unison with her.

4. Leapfrog position

Similar to the rear entry position, but instead of being on all fours, the woman lowers her torso onto the bed, while her partner penetrates her on his knees or squatting over her. This is an extremely submissive position for women, which some might find to be extremely arousing. But it's really a matter of preference.

5. Spoon split position

This sex position is a favorite of many women because it's very intimate, but also very stimulating. To perform the Spoon Split, both partners lie on their side, with the man aligning himself behind his woman. With one hand, he grasps her top leg and wraps it over his own. While he thrusts deeply, he can freely stimulate her clitoris and massage her breasts.

BEST SEX POSITIONS TO SPICE UP YOUR SEX LIFE

Great lovemaking can improve intimacy in a relationship. Besides acting as a stress reliever, making love is an important way for couples to express their love. However, in order for sex to be fun and to improve your sexual performance and confidence, there is one essential element that you need to work on. What I am referring to here is sex positioning. When boredom creeps into your bedroom, getting creative and experimenting with the different sex positions is one of the ways to break the rut.

Here are a few sex positions that can help you to rekindle the spark in your sex life

1. Reverse doggie

You adopt doggie position facing away from your woman, while she lies on her back with her legs in the air. This position allows you to control the pace of your action and makes it easier for you to stimulate her clitoris when this erogenous spot is brushed against your genitals.

2. Woman on top

a. She is facing you

She positions herself over the man's erected penis with her knees bent or on her feet flat against the man's waist. This position allows her complete movement control and gives her a lot of leeway to stimulate her clitoris by rubbing it against the man's body.

b. She is facing away from you

This position increases the chance of you hitting her elusive G-spot. At the same time, she can also use her hand to stimulate her clitoris.

c. Doing on a chair (with no arm rest) facing you or away from you. Instead of you lying on the bed, you will be leaning against a chair. She will position herself to align her "love canal" to your "little brother". This offers her the same level of sexual pleasure that she experiences when you lie on the bed with her on top.

d. Reverse frog squat

She leans forward against her knees facing away from you, adopting a squatting position like those of a frog. You lie on your back with your legs parted and penetrate her from behind. This position is ideal for those who wish for less penetration due to discomfort.

3. Reverse missionary

She lies on her back with her legs extended on the air. You face away from her, sit on her thighs and penetrate her.

The angle of penetration can be very stimulating for her

4. Modified missionary

a. Her legs extended in the air

The normal man on top position usually fails to bring a woman to reach orgasm because it is not able to provide stimulation to her clitoris and G-spot. One way to overcome this problem is to position her genitals at a higher level than your genitals so that when you penetrate her you increase the chance of hitting her G-spot. This can be done by raising her legs at 90 degrees to the air when she is lying on her back.

b. Using a pillow

Another way to raise the level of her genitals against yours is to put a pillow under the lower part of her body.

5. Modified doggie

This is quite similar to the doggie position favored by most women. She kneels on the bed and let the upper part of her body to rest on the bed (or with a pillow under the upper part of the body) with her buttocks up in the air. You then penetrate her from behind. This position can also be replicated on a big soft chair where she kneels on the seat with the upper part of her body over the back of the chair. This position is good when she is pregnant but not suitable if she has a bad neck.

6. Spoon or scissors

In this sexual position, you lie on your side with the bottom leg slightly bent. She lies on her side with her back facing you and you penetrate her with one of her legs on yours. Many people choose this position as the best way to achieve intense orgasm, possibly even multiple orgasms.

7. Semi-floating

She grabs the sides of a high stool or chair while you rest your hands under her waist to lift her off the ground. She wraps her legs around your waist and you penetrate her from behind.

8. Modified semi-floating

She faces downwards with her shoulders resting on one side of the chair and her head leaning off the side of the chair facing towards the floor. You lift both of her legs to let them rest on your shoulders (make sure her hand grabs a part of the chair to prevent her losing balance) and you penetrate her with you in a standing position. This position may not be suitable for everyone because she may feel nauseated with her head pointing to the ground.

CHAPTER FOUR
THE BEST SEX POSITION

There are lots of sex positions that you can try out in bed but most men tend to go for the ones that suit them and not their woman. To be a truly great lover you need to find the best sex positions to satisfy your woman in bed.

There are several of these that will put a smile on her face but the best two are quite the opposite of each other.

One is where she is in charge and the other is where you take control.

The woman on top is great sex position to satisfy her because not only does she get the feeling of power over you but she also controls the depth and speed of penetration. This position also makes most men last longer before ejaculating.

The best sex position to satisfy a woman sexually though is more of a sex act than an actual position. It is cunnilingus and is the one sexual act that will give her an orgasm 99 times out of 100. Cunnilingus, when performed well, can lead to multiple orgasms and even squirting female ejaculation.

While cunnilingus is the absolute best way to satisfy a woman in bed don't forget that women need more than just the sex. Unlike men sex for a woman is as much of a mental thing as a physical one. So make sure to tell her how much you fancy her and how much just looking at her turns you on.

To recap, there are loads of sex positions that can satisfy a woman in bed but none of them come even close to the pleasure that cunnilingus can give to her.

CAN SEX POSITIONS REALLY HELP YOU GET A GOOD NIGHT'S SLEEP?

If you are having trouble getting to sleep and are looking for a solution, you always think sex positions, right? Don't you? Well, OK, maybe sex positions aren't the first thing most people will think of when battling insomnia, but maybe it should be. See, sex has been proven to be a great alternative to other insomnia remedies, and is, of course, an all natural remedy! But, if you use sex as your medicine all the time, you may need to spice things ups a bit to keep that medicine bottle full! Learning and using new and different sex positions may be just the key, not only to getting a good night's sleep but also for putting a little spark back in your sex life.

Learning some new sex positions is as simple as getting copy of the Kama Sutra, watching some sex videos, or even chatting in an online forum.

You can even make some up yourself. Whatever your method it sure beats swallowing a horse's share of sleeping tablets, or brewing some chamomile tea! The main cause of sleeplessness is the brain's inability to shut down at bedtime. This is caused by over stimulus, or some kind of stressor.

Sex and the release provided by it, decompress the brain and calm the body down so it is ready for the restorative sleep it needs to remain healthy and happy.

Sleep deprivation can be dangerous to your health, so learning a few new sex positions could be the difference between being able to stave off illness or not. Sounds like a great excuse for having sex, doesn't it? Well, it's a totally legitimate reason and should be taken with some seriousness.

See, if you're over stimulate the brain before bedtime through exercise or some other endorphin promoting activity, the brain is unable to shut down resulting in the usual watching of the alarm clock until it's time to get up. Sex is the one exception because after building up the endorphins there is the release, or orgasm leaving your body and mind receptive to deep and restful sleep.

So, now when you're unable to sleep, think about sex positions and act on it. Get those endorphins ramped up then shut them right down with a nice earth-

shattering release.

You and your partner will be so happy

you did. Talk about a nice fit sleep and

waking up happy!

CHAPTER FIVE

ADVANCED SEX POSITIONS

1. The wheel barrow sex position

The Wheel Barrow position is definitely for the adventurous couples that love creative sex positions. Just like the 'wheelbarrow' races you had at school, this varied version has a definite naughty twist, making it for sex lovers who love to pound and be pounded!

To get into the wheelbarrow sex position, have him lift your pelvis as you grip his waist with your legs and support your upper body with your arms on the floor. It will definitely require stamina from both parties but a great advantage of this kinky position is the great angle it provides for g spot stimulation, as well as giving him a great view of your body. And if he's got good balance he can also stimulate your anus or clitoris.

When you get tired you can always go down on your forearms, almost like a rear aerial Pilates plank position to give your arms and shoulders a bit of a rest.

But if you love hard and fast movements, this is one of the best deep penetration positions that will appeal to those who like it rough.

2. Dancer position

Dancer Sex Position is definitely one of the most advanced sex positions because there are very few adult women who will actually be able to get into it. This tricky position requires excellent flexibility and it also helps if you are of a similar height to your partner.

To get into the dancer sex position, stand face forward, lift one leg right up over his shoulder and hold on around his waist or shoulders. Or as a variation, you can also just wrap your leg around his waist and balance on your tippy toe as he supports your weight.

Dancer sex position is fantastic for shower sex. If your man has good quad strength, he can even bounce you up and down while having the freedom to either grab on to your rear or kiss and caress you by pinning you up against the wall.

3. Viennese oyster

The Viennese Oyster is certainly one of the most creative positions that definitely requires some limbering up, but if you're flexible enough to do it, the rewards are a plenty!

To get into the Viennese Oyster position, lay back and lift both legs behind your ears giving the visual presentation of an oyster.

This may take some time getting in to as well as some practice to maintain but being one of the hardest and most advanced sex positions, it's definitely worth the time you put into preparing for it

If you can do it, it's the outright exposure and feeling of naughtiness that makes the Viennese Oyster so erotic. From this position, he can lick and suck your lady zone and can further arouse you by inserting fingers into your vagina or anus or both. Only when you are moaning for more should he penetrate and if he thrusts in hard at an upward angle this is one of the best deep penetration positions to maximize your chance of hitting your g spot.

4. Standing doggy style

Standing doggy style is great for sex on location or when you're feeling a little deviant. You will need a bench or a wall to either lean on or over to get into this naughty position. Good balance and flexible calves and thighs are also necessary to be able to withstand this position for any length of time.

A hot tip for standing doggy style is to try leaning over a bench to take some of the weight off your legs while watching yourselves in the mirror. Hot!

All of the above-advanced positions are great to work towards getting into. You can even try a bit of sexercise or different techniques to improve your flexibility and your lovemaking.

MISTAKES PEOPLE MAKE WHEN MAINTAINING THE BEST SEX POSITIONS

Most men face a common challenge when they have to decide on the best sex positions when in bed with their girl. Most of them simply fear that their girl might get bored if they repeat the same sex position every time they make love. Always keep in mind that same old always produces boring results. So they generally wonder what the best sex positions are when making love.

So, one of the best ways is to try and explain what you are not supposed to do when making sex. Most people try imitating positions they see in a number of porn movies. This is one of the main reasons why most men fail when having sex. Most inexperienced men feel the need of watching porn movies before having sex, to satisfy their girl. They just feel that porn is best as they see some of the best studs banging sexy boards..... This is what they can be named! Always keep in mind that porn movies use sex positions so viewers can see it and enjoy it. This certainly does not make it Best Positions for you!

You have to keep in mind that one of the worst sex positions is when women place her ankles on your shoulders as she might feel the pain when having sex. This is also one of the best positions that might put in all the pleasure in your sex life.

The second point to keep in mind is that you just don't have to try too hard to keep your weight away from your girl.

Sex is definitely one way in which women can get closer to her man. So if you lean on her to maintain best positions then she might love having it with you.

So, next time when you try having sex with her, please try gaining more weight so she can feel it. When having sex, most women like when she feels the weight of her man on her body. Try placing enough weight so after intercourse she might, in fact, tell you that she could feel being smushed.

Avoid grinding her pubic bone for a longer period of time as it might pain her.

Always keep in mind that in case your women is on top of you, avoid letting her do the entire job. Sex is generally considered as a passive act for most women. So in case you are motionless then she might, in fact, lose all interest in having it with you. Never destroy the entire purpose of having sex with your girl.

Maintaining one of the Best Sex Positions is possible if both of you are having an equal interest in it.

Most men also try reading books thinking they are from mars before having sex. You have to try and be an alpha male before having sex.

Best positions is when you move your girl and flip her and be a little bit aggressive. Handle her like a doll and try changing positions when having sex.

CHAPTER SIX

BEST SEX POSITIONS FOR

ORGASM

If you take a look online, you would be forgiven for thinking that there are so many amazing sex positions that you would be hard pressed to find the best sex position. If you are looking to bring your partner to orgasm, however, many of those positions may be enjoyable but not optimum for the task.

There are a couple of good sex positions that could be considered the best but only for each gender as men and women are quite different. As an aside did you know that by varying the position by just an inch can change the intensity and feeling too? This means that you should take your time and experiment with angles a bit with these positions to find what is best for you and your partner.

THE BEST SEX POSITION FOR WOMEN TO CLIMAX

For women, the 'reverse missionary' can be the best and easiest way to an orgasm. It is like the traditional missionary position except the woman is on the top rather than the man. When the woman is on top she can control the friction on her g-spot or her clitoris and has control of speed and power as well.

Usually, it is best for the women to orgasm first so once the woman is ready and aroused enough this position will allow her to climax and then you can shift to a position where the man can have control.

Where you place your legs in this position can change things a great deal depending on many physical factors, try changing your legs by spreading them or bringing them together or alternating this to find what feels best.

THE BEST POSITION FOR MEN TO ORGASM

While the missionary position is also good for guys the 'doggy style' position is often considered better because like the missionary position it gives you good control but it has a few other benefits.

Intercourse from behind while having no face to face contact (easily fixed with a mirror though) is a great position for hitting her g-spot. It also allows you full access to her sensual areas, the neck,

back, bottom and reaching around you
can also fondle the breasts and clitoris.

The other key aspect is deep penetration
which feels great for the man and for the
women, though if you are very well
endowed you may need to be careful not
to hit her cervix while doing this which
can be very painful.

THE MISTAKE COUPLES MAKE USING LOVEMAKING POSITIONS

While each position mentioned has benefits and negatives and so will every other position one problem remains that couples often fall into when trying to spice of their sex life; what happens when you try every hundred different type of position you can find in sex books and online?

In the end, they are all quite similar and you will incorporate the best ones for both of you into your lovemaking and they will become standard ... and often boring as it always feels the same.

This is why couples need to not only explore physical positions when making love but also cultivate a spirit of adventure and inventiveness into their sex lives. This is nothing dirty or sleazy it just means a few changes in the way you approach things. For instance:

Make love in a new and different place

Make love in an old place you used too but have not done for a while

Add some food into your bedroom capers

Break the routine with something exciting and different!

HOW TO GET MULTIPLE ORGASMS WITHOUT HELP OF PORN FILMS AND DIRTY SEXY PICTURES

Are you thinking of trying out a new sex position? Is the reason for this because your sex life at the minute is boring. Or, maybe you've been looking at dirty magazines filled with pictures of naked men and women in the bare flesh enjoying sex moves you never dreamed was possible, and now you're desperate for some of the action. Well why not, you're only human after all.

Some people who find they can't break the habit of looking at dirty pictures and watching porn movies, feel a sense of guilt for getting all hot and bothered under the collar, and think what they do is disgusting, and that it isn't normal, well it is, so why the panic? I'd be more inclined to worry if at the time of watching blue movies that you didn't get all sweaty and do some heavy panting.

Sex films and porn magazines can be real eye-openers, to say the least and purposely created to make the penis throb and vagina pulsate, so, if getting all hot and bothered makes you happy and you are not harming others, then continue doing what you do.

Playboy mags and porn films tend to have this magical effect on people.

They give cause for the imagination to run wild, and more often than not these people want to copy what they see, but is this a good thing? Yes of course it is, that is as long as their partner is up for it.

Warning: Before you make a move on your lover to fulfill your own desires, make sure this is what they desire too.

Communication gets you answers. If the green light to go ahead is to be given, talk things through with your boyfriend/girlfriend beforehand. If you get a no to the proposed sex position you want to try out, don't force the issue, but rather wait till the time is right to ask again.

Sexual intercourse is only good if both people come out from under the sheets satisfied. Disaster looms for any relationship when only one person leaves the bed pleased with themself. Avoid putting a strain on your relationship by making sure you know what your partner's likes and dislikes are.

Not all positions are easy to get the hang of the first time round, but with practice, the pair of you will master it. Remember, it takes two to tango, as this also applies to having sex. Both people need to make the effort for a gratifying result.

1. Happy scissors: The woman during sexual intercourse will need to raise her legs upright. The man will gently, I repeat, gently, grip each ankle spreading her legs open, parting them at 80 degrees or whatever. It's easy to get

overly excited at this point, so the man needs to be careful and in control to avoid causing pain or injury to the woman. Bruising to the ankles may happen if the man's grip is to tight, and as for parting her legs, he needs to remember they'll only open so far. This is called the happy scissor sex position, not the sad one, so take care. While the tendons of the legs pivot deep in the pelvic cavity, jostling them to and fro will subtly change sensations in the lower region for both genders.

2. Sexy stack: This includes the man kneeling down resting his buttocks on the back of his calves. The woman will sit on his lap over his erect penis with both legs straddled either side of his thighs. Start rocking and the friction will cause multiple orgasms.

3. Shake 'n' bake: If you'd like a stimulating break from intercourse, the shake 'n' bake sex move is the ideal way to do this. How it's done: The man will withdraw his penis and rest the tip on the clitoris. He'll then grip the base of

the penis and shake it from side to side so the head makes contact with the clitoris with every shake.

4. Loaded pistol: The man will sit on the bed and lean back on his arms. It's important the man gets comfortable with this sexual activity. The woman will settle over him with her legs straddled, leaning back on her arms also.

Now the pair of you will work together building up a sexy momentum by thrusting and leaning simultaneously.

This is a fantastic sex position for hitting the G-spot every go.

5. Predator: This requires the woman get on all fours so the man can enter from behind, leaving his hands free to do some stimulating handwork. This particular sex position allows the man to reach the vagina with his hands whilst his penis is still locked inside the woman from the rear. This sex move is a sort of two for the price of one, (the woman will pleasure from both angles).

6. Bend over backward: The man will lie on his back, and the woman gets on and straddle him. The woman should lean back slowly with her arms resting on the bed or floor for support. Ideal sex move for clitoral stimulation as well as deep penetration.

7. Magical: Only for the energetic: The woman lies flat on her back. The man will lift the woman's legs up to his shoulders and wrap them around his neck.

On penetration, he will hold her hips giving him more control over his thrusts. G-spot bliss!

8. Love-locked: Both people need to be on their side facing each other. His legs need to be pushed between hers, and hers wrapped around his hips as he penetrates. Fantastic sex position for clitoral stimulation!

9. Seated scissors: This move lets the woman have control in order to determine the depth and angle of penetration, as well as how much

clitoral stimulation she gets. This requires the man lying down with his knees bent and the woman straddling him. She will place one leg to the side of his hip, and the other between his legs. She will now locate the ideal spot to grind against his pubic bone while his penis is still engaged inside. This sex position is controlled more so by the woman, where she decides on the pace, depth, and the amount of pressure and friction she wants.

CHAPTER SEVEN

THE BEST SEX POSITIONS TO KEEP PREGNANCY AWAY

Best sex can always be fun and excitement, but you need to take extra control so you just don't get pregnant, especially if you are trying not to have a baby. There are a number of couples who maintain their best positions so they can have baby. For some couples, they may also try to seek the help of a fertility expert, but for some getting pregnant is an easy task. There are both positives and negatives as both couples may or may not want to have pregnancy as the outcome of their sexual intercourse. In case you are an aged couple and you certainly may never want to get pregnant then it is important that you have a better understanding of maintaining positions.

In some cases, it may, in fact, be little bit difficult to maintain as you have to ascertain that the position is best so you don't conceive.

So you have to ensure that you Don't Try these best positions if you are not trying to get pregnant. If you want to maintain best sex positions for not conceiving then avoid Missionary positions. This is the type of position in which males are generally on top of the females well secured between her legs. This should always be avoided so you don't reach maximum penetration.

This is also one way so your penis is never closer to her cervix when ejaculating.

When you go for doggy style the penis is always closer to cervix and so there are more chances of sperms being deposited near cervix. This also increases the possibilities of conceiving, so in case you are planning not to get pregnant then please avoid this best sex positions. If you are looking for not getting pregnant then avoid scissors. In this position, both male and female are generally on the opposite sides of each other. This is also one best position if both want to touch each other's sex organs.

If you want to maintain best sex positions to avoid pregnancy then maintain L position. This position is best created when you join your hips with your partner's thighs. These are some of the best sex position if you want to conceive or not, but you have to keep in mind that these are just not foolproof methods. Sex is just about birth control, but it more about fun and excitement. Maintain your best sex positions such that you get more fun and excitement with your partner in the bed.

BEST SEX POSITIONS FOR COUPLES LOOKING FOR THE G-SPOT

Are you interested in the best sex positions for couples? More specifically those focusing on the g-spot? If for some strange reason you have never heard of the g-spot, the g-spot is a term used to describe the area of a women's vagina that when stimulated properly can lead to very powerful orgasms.

If you are looking for some new and best sex positions for couples to try then I would highly suggest positions that can lead to g-spot orgasms. Watching and experiencing your lady have g-spot orgasms is highly arousing for men as well.

Three of the best sex positions for couples that you can try for g-spot stimulation are the cowgirl, accordion and the ever faithful doggy style.

1. Cowgirl position: This is becoming one of the best sex positions for couples and has the women on top of the man, kneeling and leaning forward towards him. The man, while on his back, should

try and tilt his pelvis forward as much as possible. The tilting of the pelvis, along with her being on top, allows for the proper angle to help stimulate her g-spot. To changes, this position slightly have her brace herself with her feet instead of her knees. This is also known as the Aggressive Cowgirl

2. Accordion position: This is one of the relatively unknown best sex positions for couples that also has the women on top. The man is sitting semi cross-legged and the women then sit on the man's penis

while facing away from him. The women then lean forward with her hands touching the ground and then makes a back and forth motion. The women is now able to control the angle and degree of penetration allowing for excellent g-spot stimulation. Making this one of the best sex positions for couples looking for g-spot pleasure.

3. Doggy style: This position is very common and is by far one of the best sex positions for couples. What most do not know is that the position is great for

stimulating the g-spot. With the women crouching on all fours, legs slightly apart, the man enters from behind. This position stimulates the g-spot while also allowing for deeper penetration if desired

If g-spot stimulation is what you and your partner would like to explore than I highly recommend trying all three of these best sex positions for couples. Experiment and communicate with each other and before you know it these will be a part of your repertoire.

MAINTAIN THE BEST SEX POSITION TO STRIKE THE G-SPOT!

Yes, it is true as there certainly are a number of ways of having good sex and then you certainly have a number of best positions that might satisfy both of you. You have to discover the best sex position for you can help to hit the G-spot. It is of prime importance for you to understand that having sex with your partner for three to four minutes is never going to satisfy her. You have to, in fact, try to read and understand this book for best sex position and try to implement them when making sex with your partner more often. It is very much important that you try and communicate with your partner so you are sure to be present on the same page and understand that everything is just working out fine.

You have to keep in mind that the G-spot is a region that is present behind the pubic bone and the moment this is stimulated it allows your women to experience a mind-blowing orgasm. So before you actually get inside your women it is important that you try and play with her for sometime. This simple exercise might also help in discovering her G-spot and its exact location. Exploring is a good option but when trying out Best Sex Positions you certainly have to be very gentle to her. When having best sex with your women there certainly are a number of best sex positions available that might help in reaching the G-spot climax that you are in fact looking for.

When you are making use of standard missionary style, you just need to ensure that you lift your girl's hips to a much higher elevation so you can enjoy maximum penetration inside her giving her more pleasure. When on top you should also try to put more amount of weight on her so she can feel you. There are a number of men who try having sex without actually shifting their weight on her with an aim to maintain Best Sex Positions You have to keep in mind that most women enjoy weight, so don't just keep it to yourself. Always bear in mind that women like having their men on top of them and when they feel the pressure of pelvic against her, this might be the right time to hit the G-spot.

When working for best position it is important that you try out different positions discussed and then decide on which is the one that might stimulate her. When having sex with your women it is important that you try and locate her G-spot soon or else she might just lose all interest in having it with you. Try to increase her intensity by using the best sex position which she is comfortable with.

CHAPTER EIGHT
ORAL SEX POSITIONS

Oral sex is a fun and exciting part of any relationship, but would you like to know more positions to try to make it feel even better?

There are many different positions, and after mastering these maneuvers, use your creativity to make up your own! If so, then read these new, and sexy positions to try with your partner tonight!

Comfortable positions

If you take a long time to give your partner oral sex and would like to be comfortable while doing it, try laying on your back and having your partner leaning over the bed.

Not only is this comfortable for both of you, but it allows your partner to work on you without any restrictions. It is also comfortable for the woman to be on her knees.

The favorite position

The sixty-nine position seems to be a long time favorite oral sex position that isn't going away any time soon! Why should it when it allows no restrictions for the woman to work, and gives the man the view of his dreams?

This is also a great position because it allows both of you to be doing the oral sex at the same time, which doesn't make one partner feel like they are doing all the work.

This position may seem awkward at first, but trust me, you'll both like it!

The sexy position

Now, these are more for show than they are pleasure sometimes because you are so focused on holding your pose! Women can try straddling her partner's face. This may seem awkward for her, but he loves it. You will be able to focus more on the pleasure if you have something to hold on to, such as a bedpost or the back of the couch.

These oral sex positions are simply a starting point. Once you get the hand of it you can create your own positions that feel the best to you.

TIPS ON ORAL SEX

Oral sex is something every woman wants, which means that it is extremely important for you to get tips on how to perform a good oral sex if you want to please her in bed.

There are more than 8,000 nerve endings on a woman's clitoris, which makes it the most sensitive part of a human body. This explains why women can easily achieve orgasms just from oral sex itself. Therefore, with something that sensitive, you better make sure that you know what you are doing before you go poking around with your tongue.

Let us just discuss some of the tips on oral sex which can make you a better licker:

1. Get her into the right mood. This is something that you need to know before we can get down to the various oral sex techniques. Women take time to get turned on, whereas men tend to rush for intercourse. If you wish to let your woman enjoys the sexual experience, you need to focus more on foreplay and set up the right mood for her. Create the sexual anticipation and desire, and she will give you the cue to go down on her once she is ready.

2. Control your strokes. The pace of your strokes can determine whether she will enjoy the oral sex that you give her. The safest bet is to start your stroke slowly. Ask her how she feels, and how you are able to improve your strokes. As you see she is getting turned on, you can start to increase the pace of your strokes gradually.

3. Make use of different oral sex positions. As there are different positions for intercourse, it applies to oral sex too.

Different position can trigger different sensation, and it will be fun for you to try it out with your lover. A few common positions are the "69", Doggie Style and the Scissors.

It is definitely well worth your time to master the art of oral sex if you want your lover to achieve orgasms. Performing oral sex on women is definitely a much better and faster way to let them achieve mind-blowing orgasms, as long as men know how to do it right.

Do you know that 81% of women regularly achieve orgasms from cunnilingus when compared to only 25% from traditional vaginal penetration? This gives you a more compelling reason why you must master the art of cunnilingus if you want to please your lover.

ORAL SEX POSITIONS FOR MAXIMUM PLEASURE

If you need to add some spice to your sex life, try the different oral sex positions. Oral sex can be a wonderful foreplay to get your partner aroused. You can even take it to the full extent and get an orgasm through oral sex.

Here are some positions you can try:

When you are giving her oral sex, try raising her hips a little. You can do this by putting a pillow under her waist or making her lie down on the edge of her bed while you play with your tongue and tease her vagina into ecstasy. Having her pelvis tilted at an angle will make it easier for you to continue in that position without straining your neck when she is nearing a climax!

When you have her on the edge of the bed, try wrapping her leg around your shoulder at a raised angle. This will open up her vagina and give you more access.

Don't zero in on the clitoris at once. Initially, go for long strokes with your tongue. While you are doing this, don't forget to use your hands also. You can stroke her thighs and her tummy all the while.

You can even get her to squat at while you have a go. Just make sure she is balancing herself on her knees and you are under her, but not bearing her whole weight!

Another interesting position is to have her upside down so that she is balancing herself on her arms and is supported by either you or some furniture. You might need some practice for this, but the rush of blood to the head this achieves will make you more than happy! This will put you in a better position to get her aroused. You can try all these positions at the same time or just one at a time. Try these oral sex positions and get her screaming for more!

MASTERING ORAL SEX POSITIONS

I know there are thousands of women in the world who enjoy giving their men oral sex! Why shouldn't you? It's nice to hear him moan and see him move around the bed as you're stimulating his manhood with your tongue. Just make sure he's STD free because there is nothing worse than getting an STD in the mouth. Before I get in depth about all the positions you can try, let me enforce a rule in oral sex.

Don't ever bite his penis because that is very painful for men. How would you feel if he bit your vagina during cunnilingus? I know you wouldn't like that. The same applies to men because that part of their body is very sensitive.

Here are oral sex positions you should try with your partner:

1. Squatting

What is sexier than giving your partner head while you're squatting? Most men love it when their women squat in front of them and start sucking on their penises. You should grab his nipples during this session because this is just as sensational for him as it is for you.

2. Laying down

I think it's very romantic for a man to go down on his woman while she's lying down. Lick her clitoris slowly and then pick up speed. Even lick it in circular motion. Doing so will drive her crazy and make her climax quicker. Women take longer to come than men do, that's why you have to put in more effort when you're trying to accomplish this.

3. Sitting down

Most women wish their men would open their legs, and begin to lick their vagina at a random time. Well, luckily there are a few men who are willing to do that. Give him a signal by wearing sexy clothes and sitting with your legs open. Any man with common sense will know what you want.

4. Lying on your stomach

If you like to try new positions, I'd recommend you to try this one! Why? Because you'll have more fun receiving oral sex lying on your belly. Trying new positions will add more excitement and make you look forward to giving and or receiving head.

I guarantee you these positions will make you enjoy the art of having sex and form a closer bond with your mate. Why continue to try the same, boring positions when you can try new and creative ones? Keeping your options open will make you a better lover and enhance your skills in the bedroom!

THE MOST SCINTILLATING ORAL SEX POSITIONS

There are a number of positions you can try for orals sex. Here are a few we like. Remember every woman is different. You will have to explore all your options before you hit on the one that is just right for you.

The best and the most popular position for oral sex is, of course, the 69 position. In this position, both your sensitive areas are open to each other and you can have the time of your life pleasuring your partner.

You can even try a variation of the doggy style for maximum pleasure. In this position, your partner will be balancing herself on her arms and knees, while you lie on your back, just between her legs. This position is the best for oral sex because it leaves her vagina wide open and lets you use your fingers to caress her all the time you are sending her to heaven with that tongue!

The edge of the bed is the best position to drive her to the edge of sanity with your fingers and tongue! In this position, you kneel on the ground while she is resting on her back on the bed or chair. Spread her legs wide while you pleasure her. You can even use a hot and cold tongue to add the extra pleasure to your moves. Just suck on some ice or sip on hot water before delving into her.

You can even alternate between the two for maximum impact.

Another hot position to go for is to have her riding you. As long as she is not suffocating you, you have perhaps one of the best positions in which you can pleasure her. Spread her legs on both your sides and have her balance herself on her knees. Position your mouth well and then, drive her nuts! Try out these oral sex positions. And yes - keep those windows soundproofed!

SOME BENEFITS AND DISADVANTAGES ORAL SEX POSITIONS

When we think of good sex, we probably think of multiple positions and techniques. What is strange is that we do not apply this same thinking to other kinds of sex. In fact, all other kinds of sex have many different positions. For guys varying the positions for oral sex can give you a great added thrill for both you and her.

One of the most common moves is the 69 and most people are familiar with it, so you can have some fun with it by alternating from being on the top to being on the bottom. Secondly, by placing a cushion under her hips you can angle them upwards to make it easier to access her clitoris. If she likes this feeling, she can move the pillow further up (To the small of her back) and this will angle her clitoris downwards, giving her different stimulation.

One of the fun oral sex positions is for her to be on top. You will want to reverse the previous technique and have the pillow under your hips. Experiment with some angles as some will allow her to go deeper than others. With her on top, she also has more control over her own pleasure and can grind her hips against your mouth and tongue. From this position, it is easy to access her perineum and anus if she likes those kinds of stimulation too.

As she gets more excited she can increase the thrill by raising to sitting position (Make sure she takes some weight on her legs or agree on a way to signal if it is uncomfortable). This elevated position allows her to really grind her hips and bring herself more quickly to orgasm.

If the straddle is too much for you, then move her to a standing position. This has some benefits and disadvantages.

The benefit is that this oral sex position gives you easy access to both the clitoris and even the G-spot. The big problem is that your neck muscles are relatively weak, so it can be tough for her to get the right amount of pressure to really have an intense orgasm. Therefore what I recommend is to get her to lean back against the wall. This has two advantages: it allows you to lean into her, using stronger muscles to lock your head and it allows you more access to her erogenous zones.

Of course, no oral sex positions guide would be complete without doggy-style. This can be a great addition to oral sex as it gives the guy so many options about what to stimulate. By mixing oral sex and perineum/anal play, you can really give her a range of great feeling.

Like other kinds of sex play, variation and constant surprise are the most important things. These techniques are great for helping women to have their first orgasm or giving her yet another one. Make sure that you surprise her as much as possible, changing the angles, positions, strength, and frequency all the time. Once you find one that brings her to orgasm, stick to it and watch her go wild.

WAYS TO PLEASE YOUR MAN WITH ORAL SEX

If you want to know how powerful oral sex is, ask any man how they felt when they got their first blowjob and you will be amazed at the responses.

Awesome! Out of this world! Mind-blowing! These are some the most likely words they will use to describe how they felt! It, therefore, makes perfect sense to start learning how to please a man with oral sex. You need to know how to take him there. Here are seven ways to please your man with oral sex... Read on;

1. Make him comfortable. The first and the most important thing you need to remember is that your man has to be comfortable before giving him oral sex. This will keep him at ease and ensure

that he has your full concentration. Ensure that you do all you can to make him feel relaxed so that he can take his time to reach orgasm. In other words, don't make him feel like you're in a rush.

2. Let him assume the perfect position. Let your man get in the perfect position. This also contributes to his relaxation levels. You can place a pillow under his butt so that his penis is in a raised position. The higher the penis, the easier it is for you to access it which ultimately means it will be easier to pleasure him.

The other perfect position you can let your man take is the standing position while you kneel down. Remember oral sex is not all about his genital. It extends to his other erogenous zones, so work them too.

3. Use your tongue. While you will use your mouth to give him most of the oral sex, you can use your tongue to increase his pleasure. Start by licking his groin area up and down while moving to his nipples and other parts slowly. Before

you work his penis, lick his inner thighs and his perineum as well.

4. Watch for his body language. If you want to know how to please a man with oral sex, you need to listen and watch the way he reacts when you work on certain parts of his body. This will help you know which points give him pleasure. If he moves his body when you suck his balls, for instance, you may want to be sure you give them some attention too. Listening to his body also helps you know which sequence to

follow when giving him oral sex. You may have to interchange the licks between his points of pleasure and other parts that are not as sensitive.

5. Add some sex toys. Yes! Sex toys can be can an incredible addition to oral sex if you're serious about pleasing your man. Men climax much faster than women, thus bringing sex toys in between oral sex can prolong the amount of time he takes to reach orgasm. Don't use a very large sex toy; use something small that can be easily

handled so you remain in control. You can use a sex toy to tease his inner thighs while licking his balls or his penis.

6. Increase the momentum as things heat up. To make sure your man gets the ultimate pleasure, increase the tempo as he gets more and more engrossed in the act. You can prolong the amount of time his penis or balls remain in your mouth. Watch for his reactions as he gets closer to orgasm and focus on the parts that he derives much pleasure from. This will

make both of you prepared for his orgasm.

7. Don't relent. Don't stop what you're doing even when he just about to hit the climax because that's how you please a man. Instead, get prepared for the moment. Don't be surprised if he doesn't come since your goal was to make him feel good and not a reflection of what you can do with your mouth.

Giving a man some oral pleasure can not only turn out to be the sexiest and intimate thing you could do, but one of the easiest way to please your man as well. Remember that what makes oral sex pleasurable is the attitude you portray to your partner.

CONCLUSION

Young people are always active and energetic in their relationships and term their love life 'booming' and 'spicy'. However, this does not mean that senior people who are not termed 'young' anymore cannot enjoy their relationships at this golden age. Most of the senior aged people sometime term their relationships as boring because their relationships have been progressing at the same rate for many years.

They do not introduce anything new sex positions in their relationships fearing that it might strain it. However, this doesn't always have to be the case. Seniors can also spice up their relationships with a few tips and tricks in this book with any harm.

If you're looking for some easy sex positions but still want to make her orgasm and give her some amazing sexual experiences, then you'll want to read this book again and again.

Many people think that just because a specific sex position is easy, means it's not very effective or capable of leading to massive pleasure for both of you. This simply isn't true. Learn different easy sex positions and also some very simple tricks and tips to make them a lot more stimulating.